One in Ten Thousand

Written and Illustrated by: Christy L. Ott, MD, MSc, FAAP

Cover Page by Calvin Ott, Artist and Musician

Parson's Porch Books

To order additional copies of this book, contact:

Parson's Porch Books
1-423-475-7308
www.parsonsporch.com

Parson's Porch Books is an imprint of Parson's Porch & Company (PP&C) in Cleveland, Tennessee. PP&C is an innovative non-profit organization which raises money by publishing books of noted authors, representing all genres. All donations from contributors and profits from publishing are shared with the poor.

Dedication

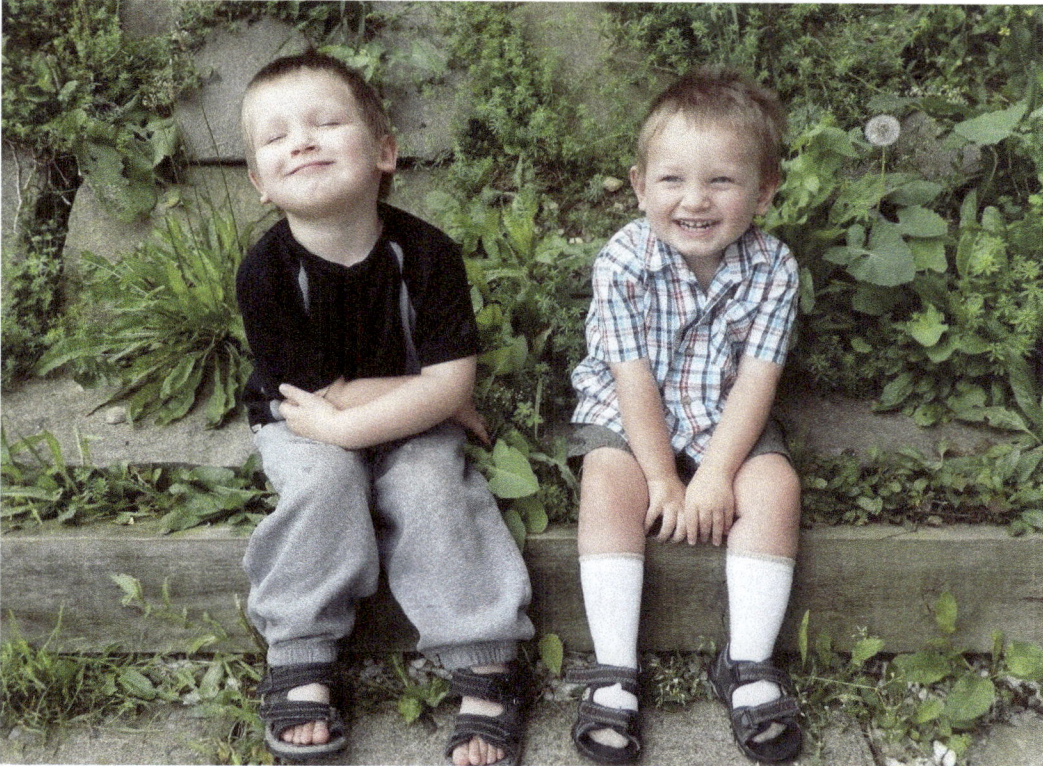

This book is dedicated to: Kalen (L) and Kyan Kulas (R) and family. Thank you for being an inspiration. Children like you give me a desire to work harder everyday to learn innovative ways to heal, cure, and treat patients.

Thank you to my mommy, Lucy Mae Ott (looking on from Heaven) who taught me that there is nothing I cannot do or become. Thank you to my father, Jerry Ott, Sr. who is always there to listen and support, step-mom Elease Parker Ott, brothers Jerry Jr., Alvin, Philemon, sister Celeste and extended family and friends. Thank you to Family Health Services in Chattanooga, TN and Drs. Shaw, Hubbard, & Brooks who support and encourage me, and to our staff who help us daily to accomplish our aims to provide excellent healthcare in Hamilton County. I would like to express my sincere gratitude to Dr. Cathy Stevens from the Medical Genetics department at Children's Hospital at Erlanger for her support, her time, and her advice. Thank you to my pastor Dr. Joe McKeever who still mentors me long after I've grown up and moved away and to his lovely wife Mrs. Margaret (who also awaits us in Heaven). Thanks also to Karen Barbour for sparking a great idea. Thanks to all of my teachers, attendings, classmates, mentors, to 800 Collective in Chattanooga, Children's Hospital at Erlanger, and most importantly, thanks to God from who all blessings flow.

Foreword

Dear Parent,

Receiving a diagnosis of SMA can feel devastating, hopeless, and as if your entire world has ended. There are thousands of us who have felt that exact same way, and we are here to say that there is LIFE beyond diagnosis. There is HOPE beyond grief, and you will feel TRUE HAPPINESS, again.

Prepare to live life with more APPRECIATION than you have ever felt before! You will learn more from your child than you could ever teach him/ her. Open your heart to the possibility that you and your child are both equally blessed. He/ she may be ONE IN TEN THOUSAND, but being his/ her parent is truly the best!"

-Sierra Kulas, *Mother of Kalen & Kyan who are both children with SMA Type 2*

They say that I'm **SPECIAL**, one of a kind, *lucky*, and **unique**.

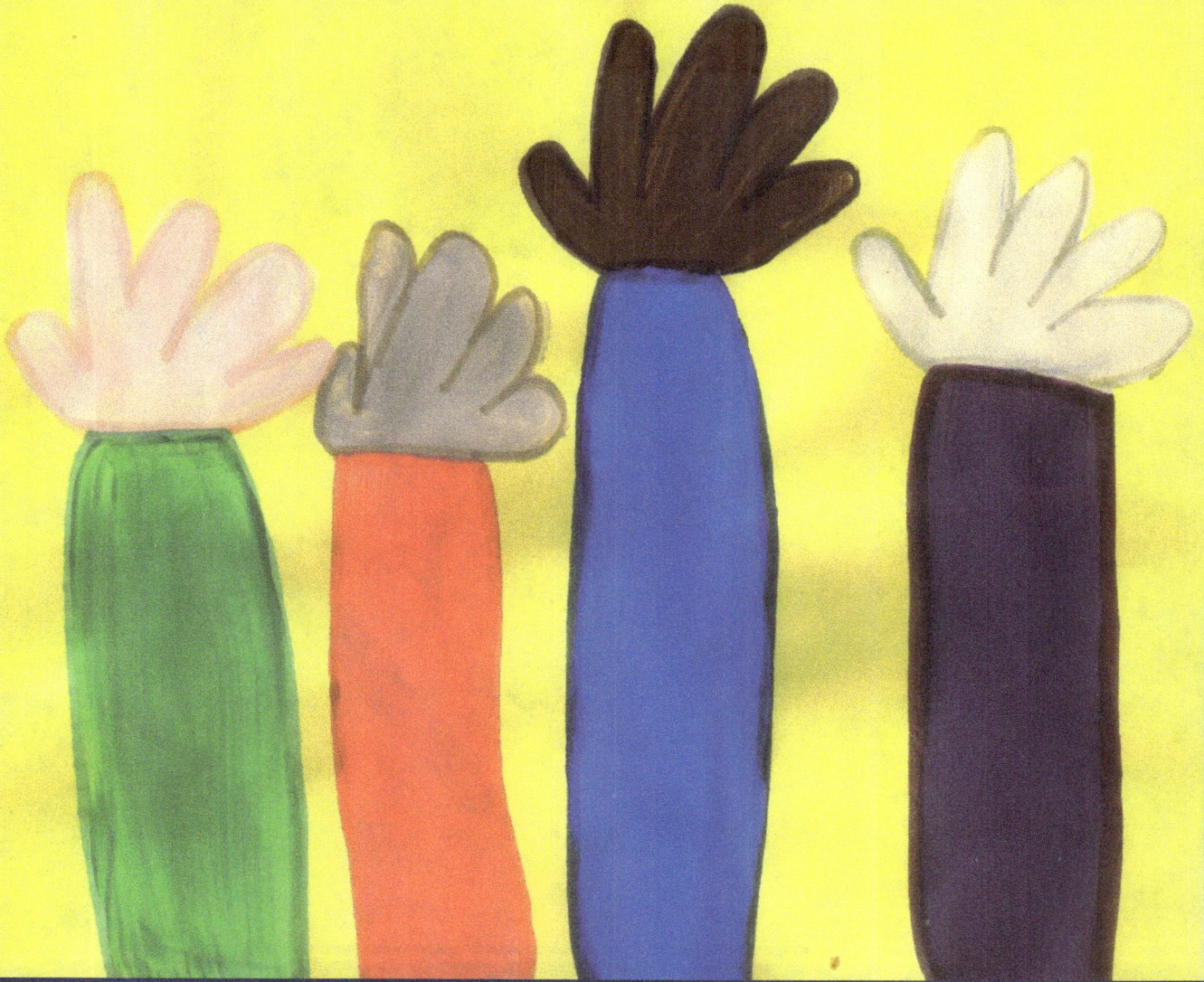

Well, that is one statement I would like to critique!

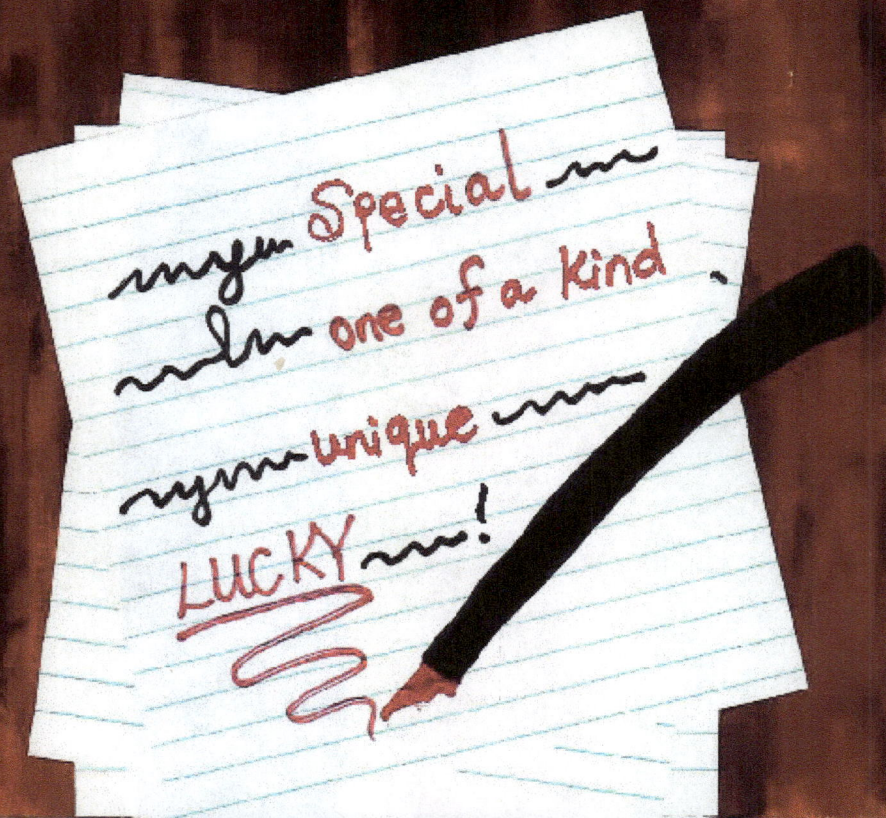

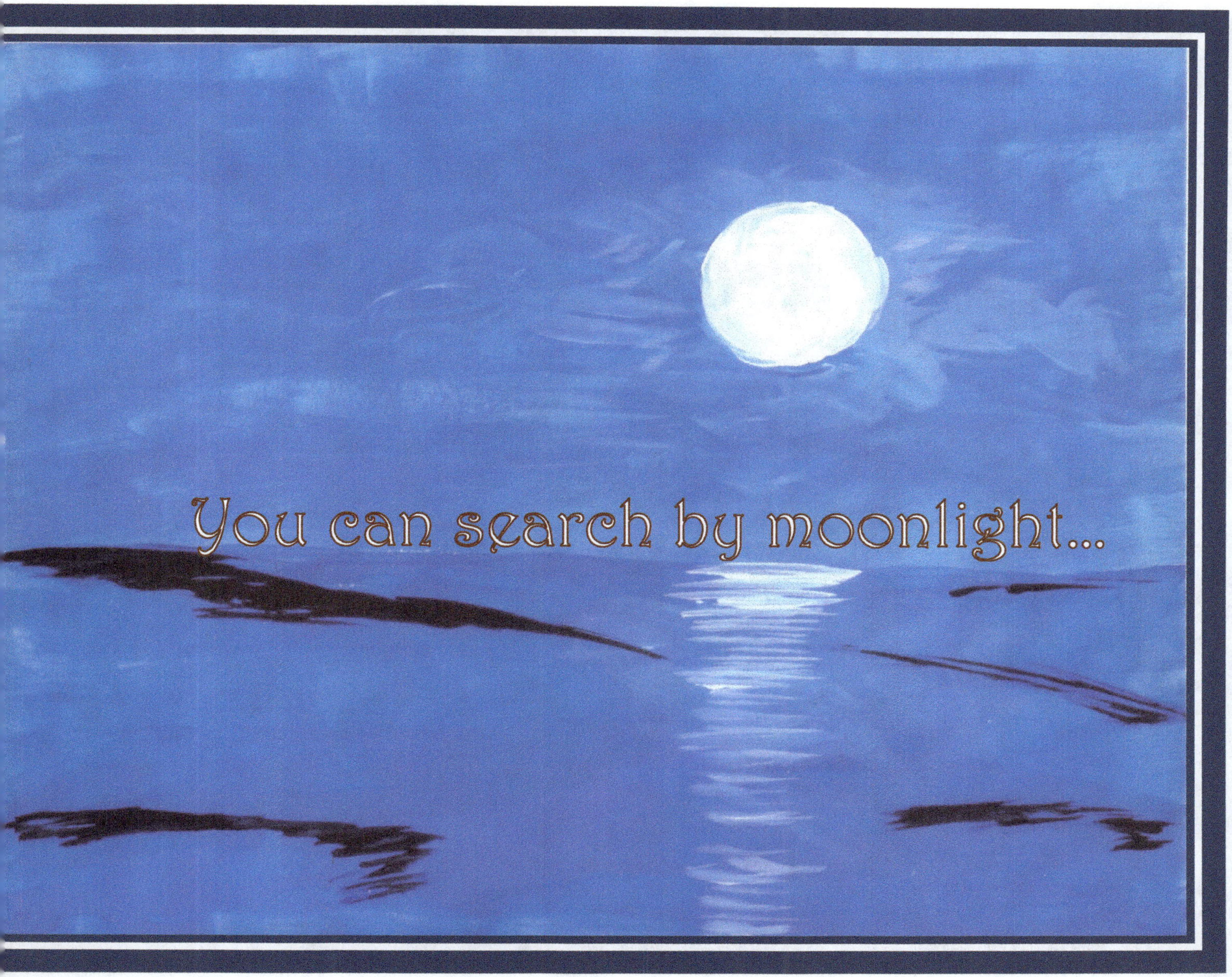

You can search by moonlight...

...Or under the sun.

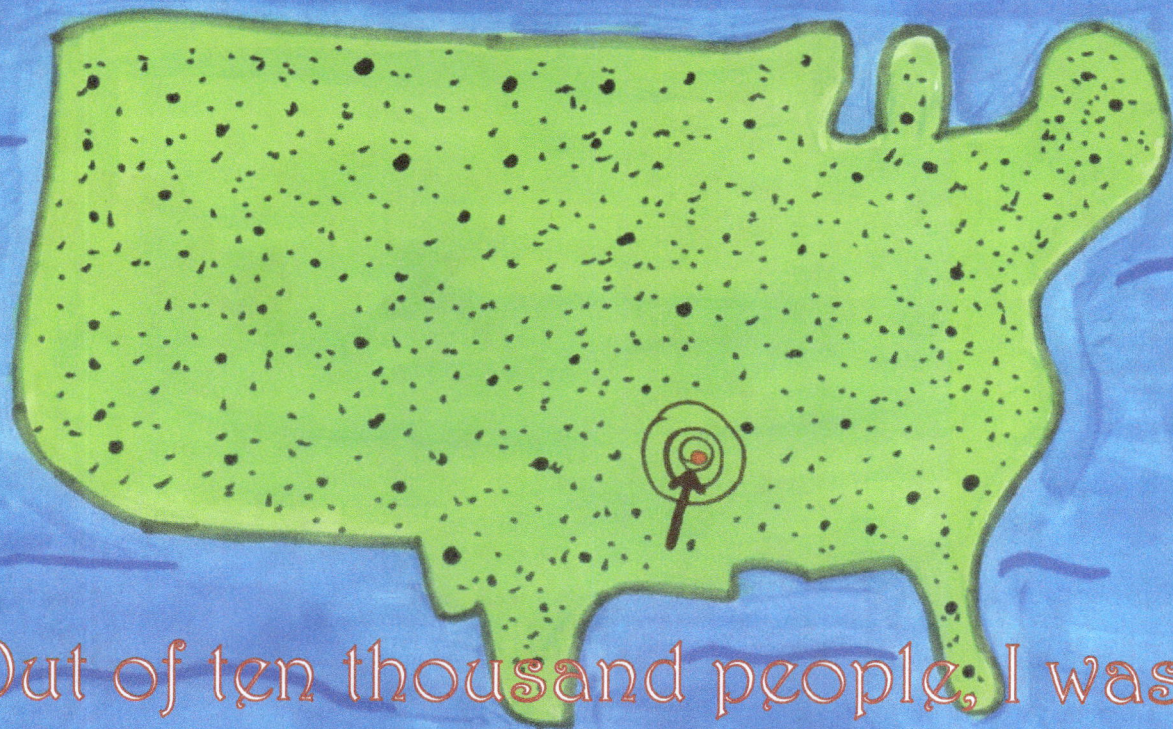

Out of ten thousand people, I was the one!

Some people are lucky to win prizes, money, and fame!

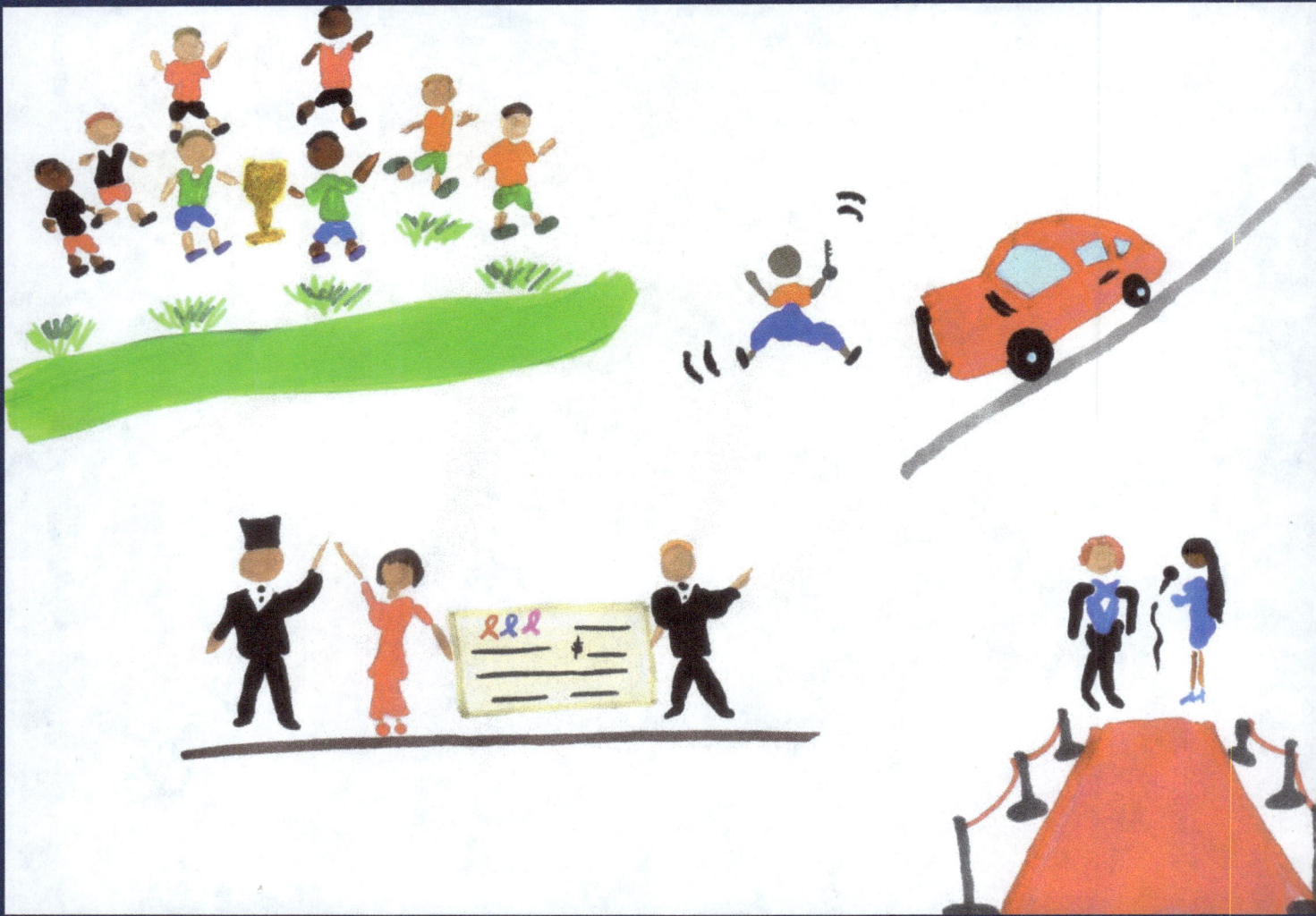

However, I won a condition, and I can't pronounce its name.

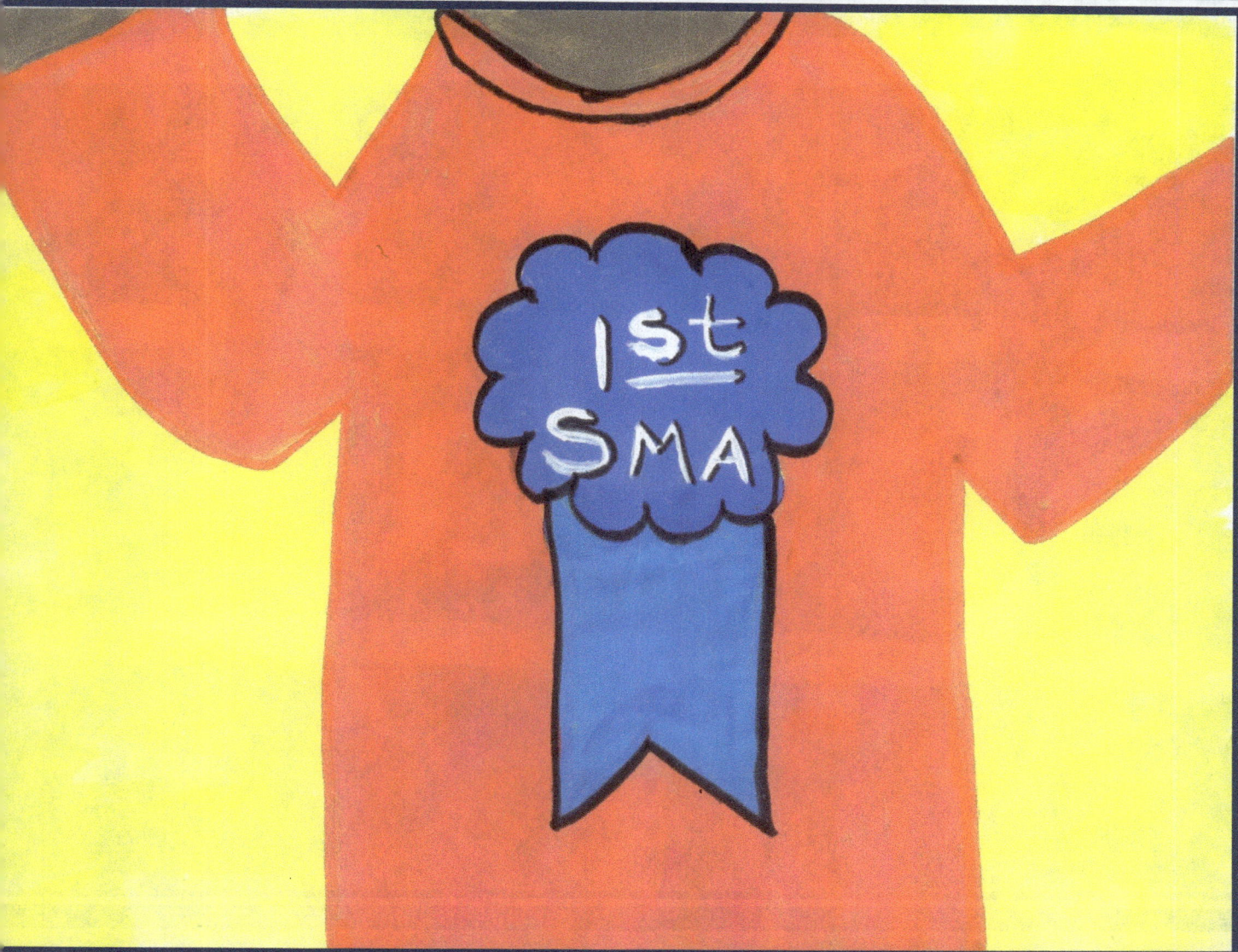

Spino-Musica... No spina musta trophy... Oh SMA! Just learn the initials. It's easier to say!

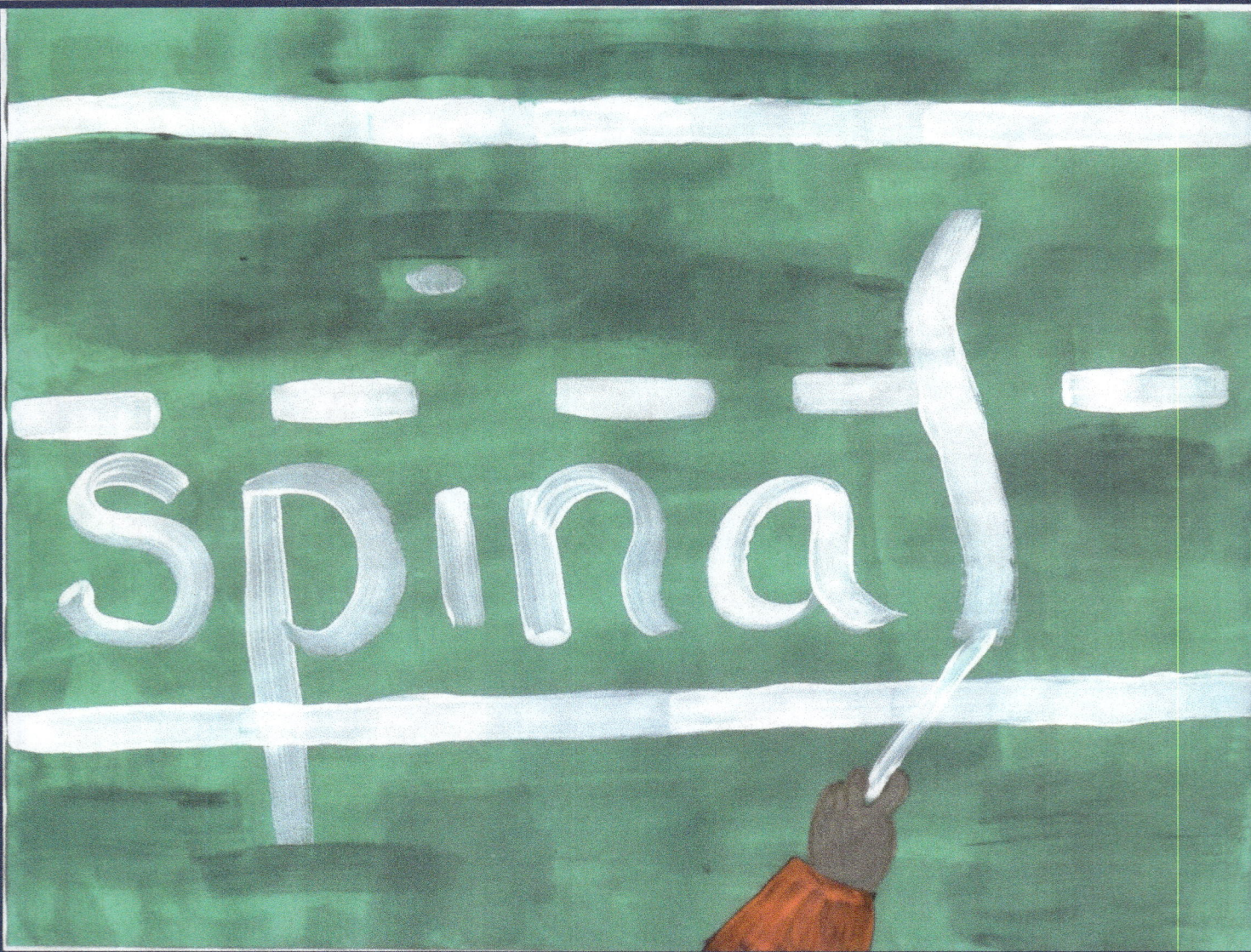

Honestly, it's a relief to
know what it's called.
At 9 months old, I could
not scoot or crawl.
Sometimes, I don't have
energy to move at all!

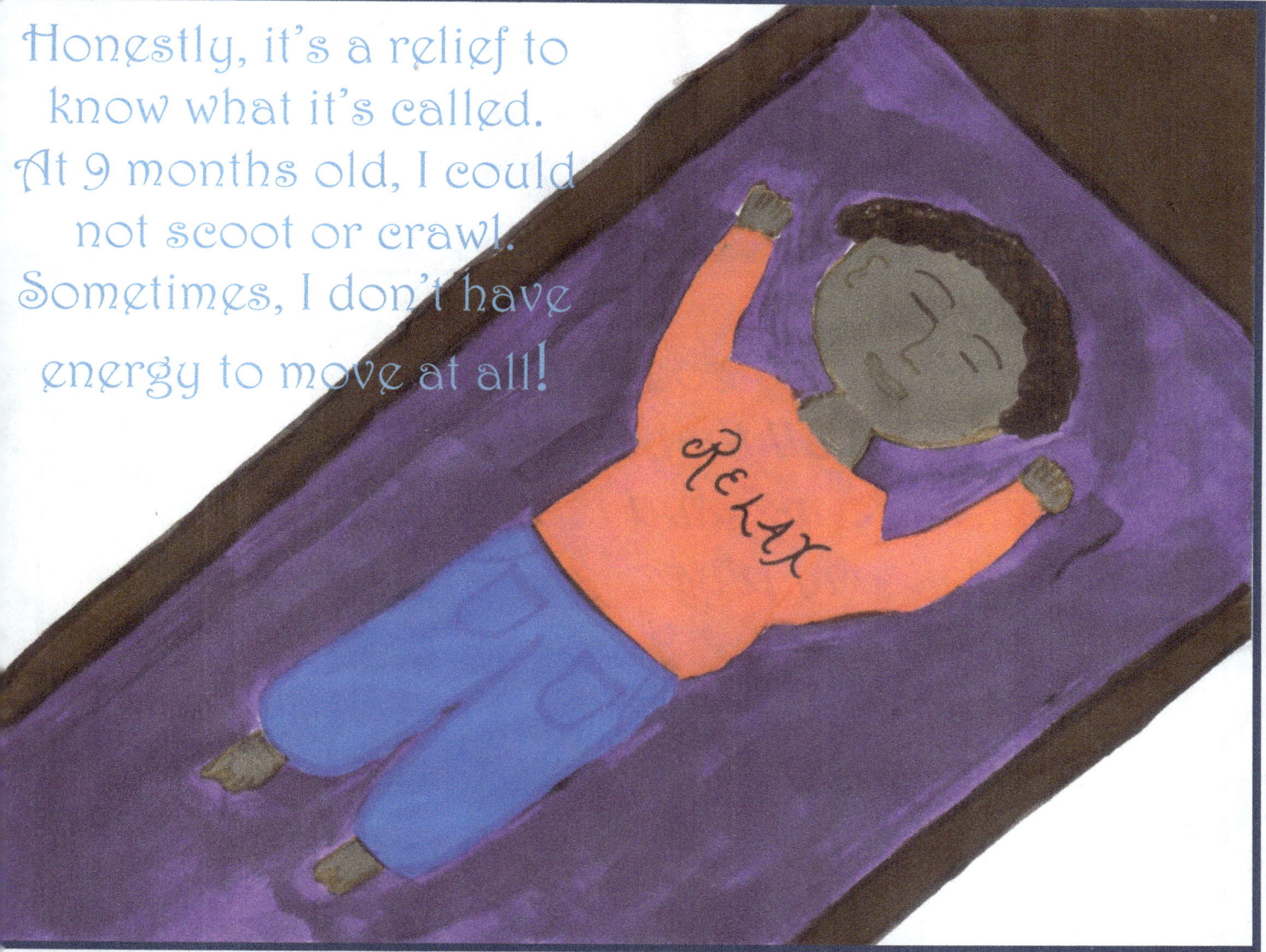

When I sit on the curbside and watch other kids run and race,
My parents gaze at the expression on my face;

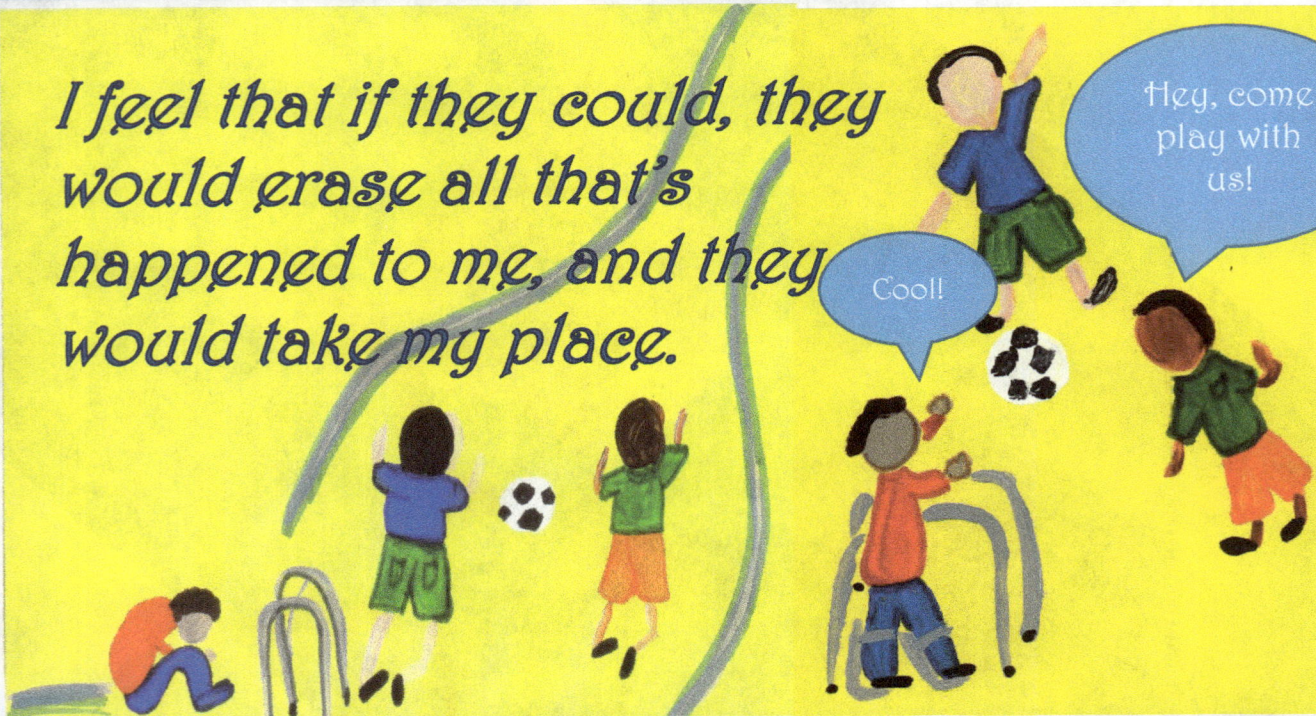

Even breathing has become a difficult task.
If I could meet God, I'd have questions to ask.

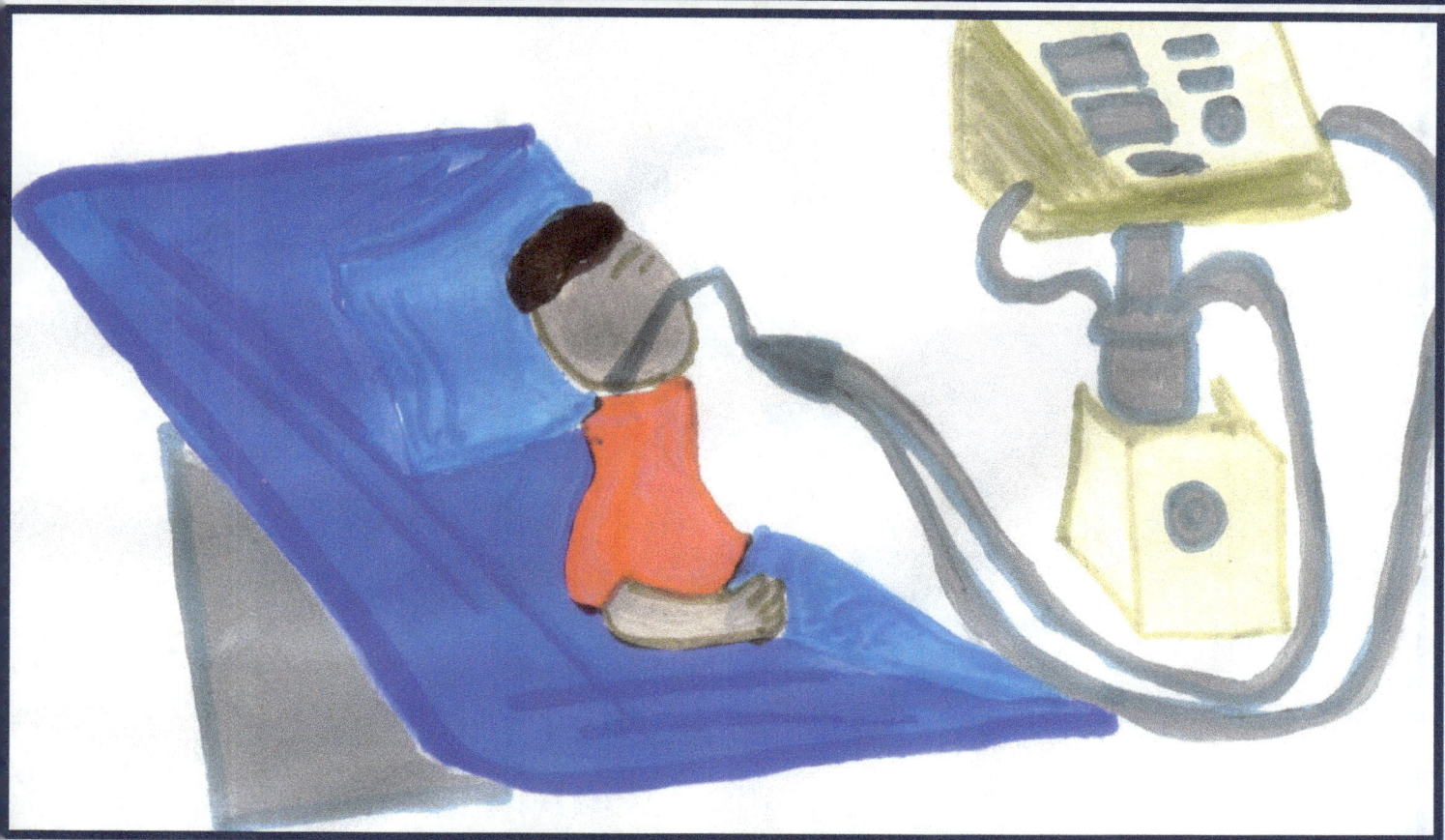

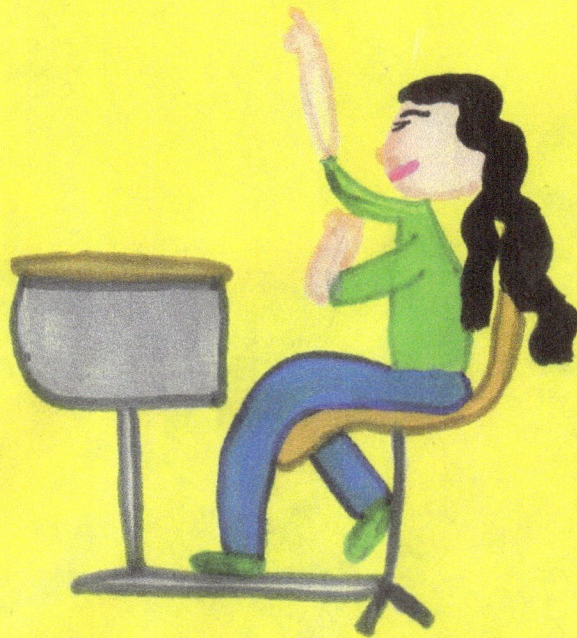

I wonder and ponder, "How could this be?
If God is so perfect, how could He do this to me?"

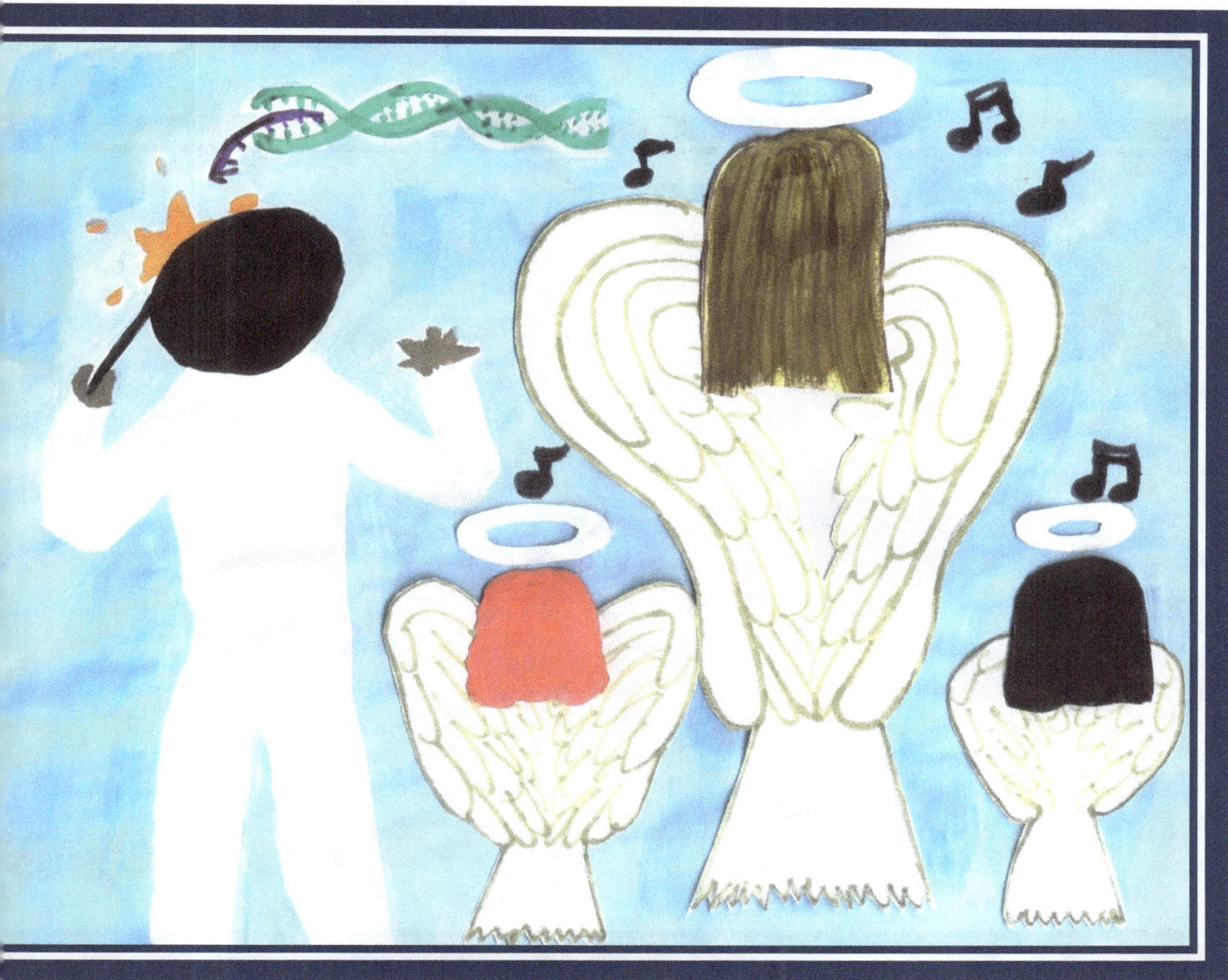

"Did the angels distract Him while He was creating?"

"Did He order my genes and get tired of waiting?"

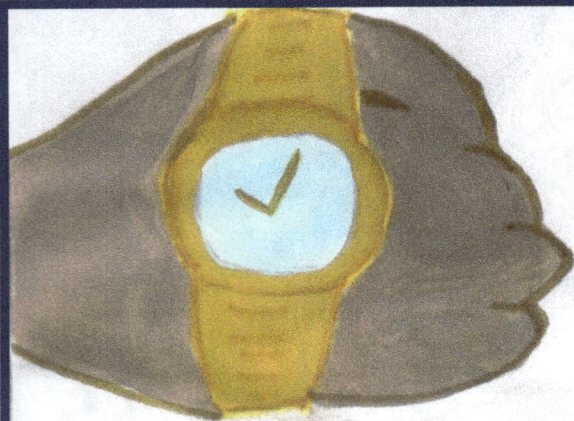

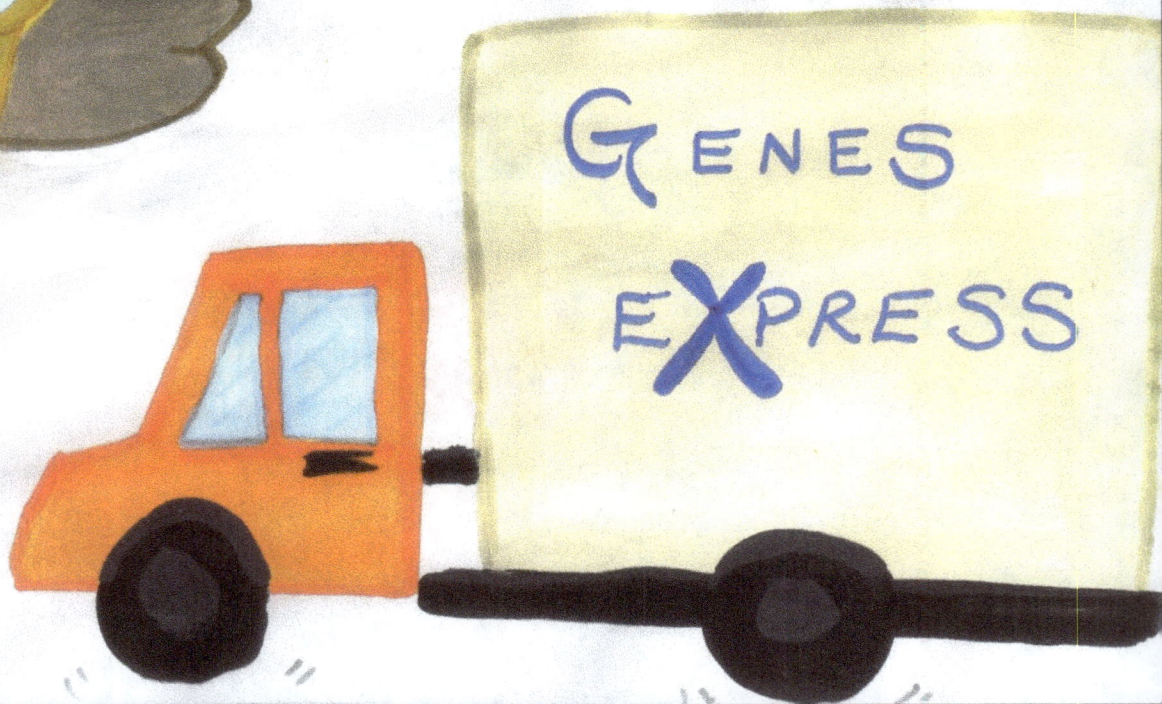

"Did He skip a step or feel weak and tired that day?

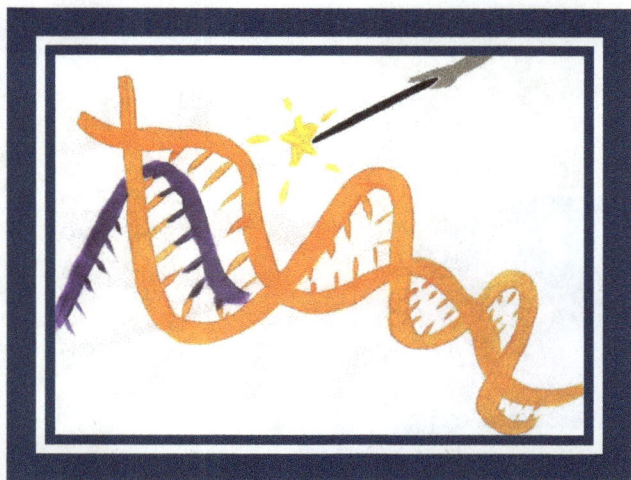

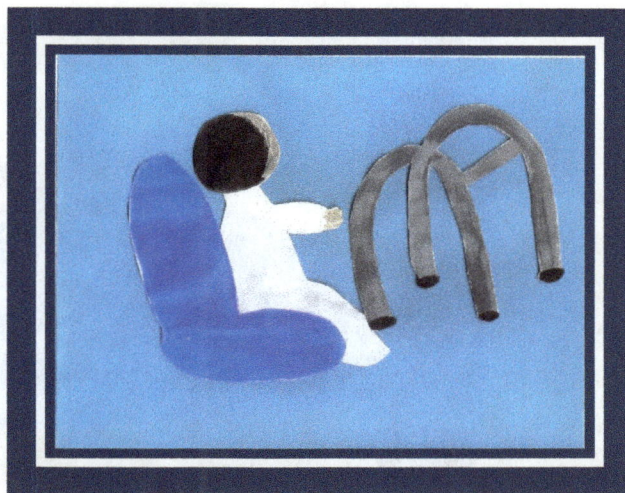

Hey, do you think that maybe God has SMA?"

Just kidding 🙂

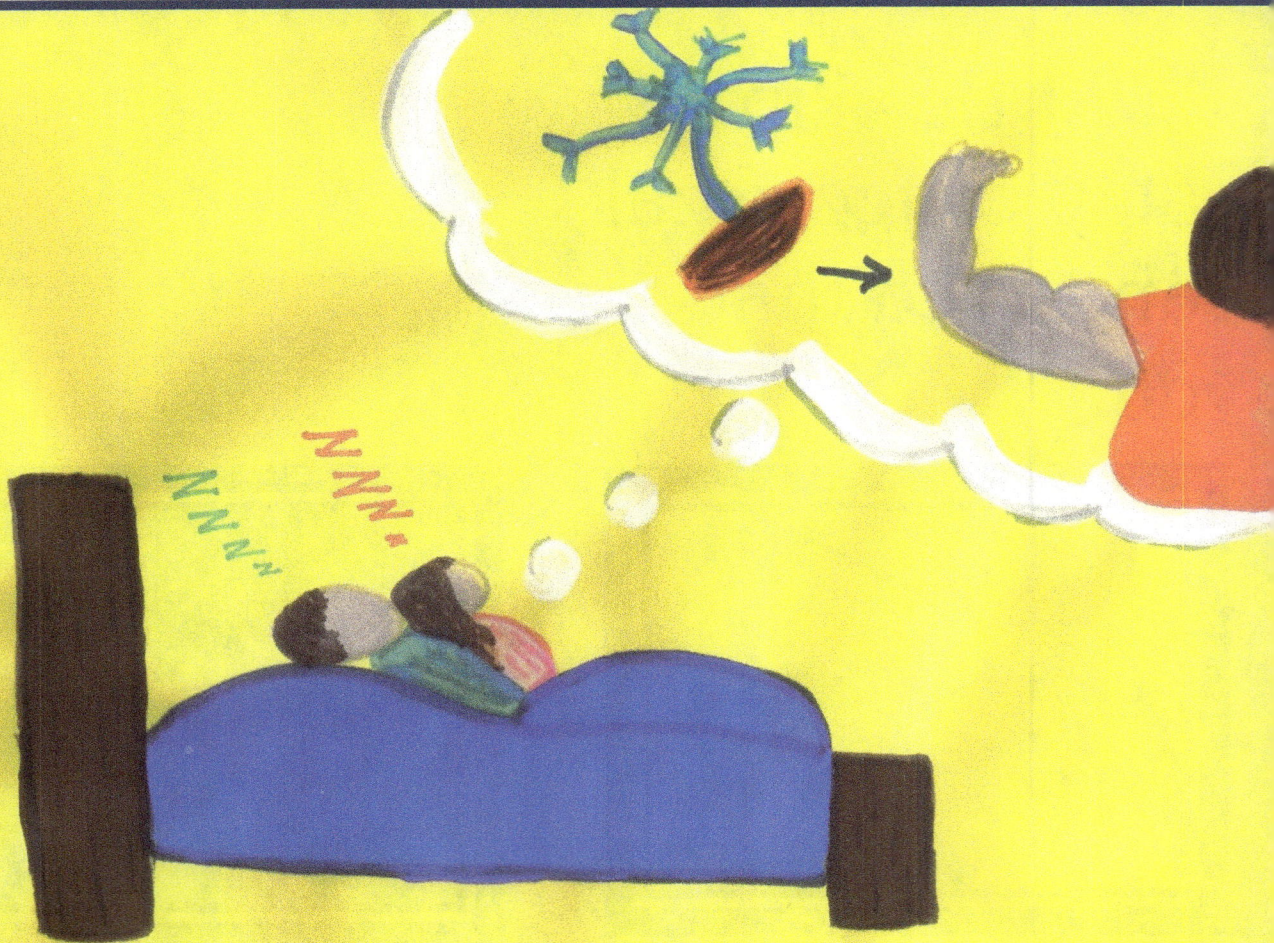

Daddy and Mommy love me so much, and it does
truly seem that finding a cure for my weakness is
their wildest dream.

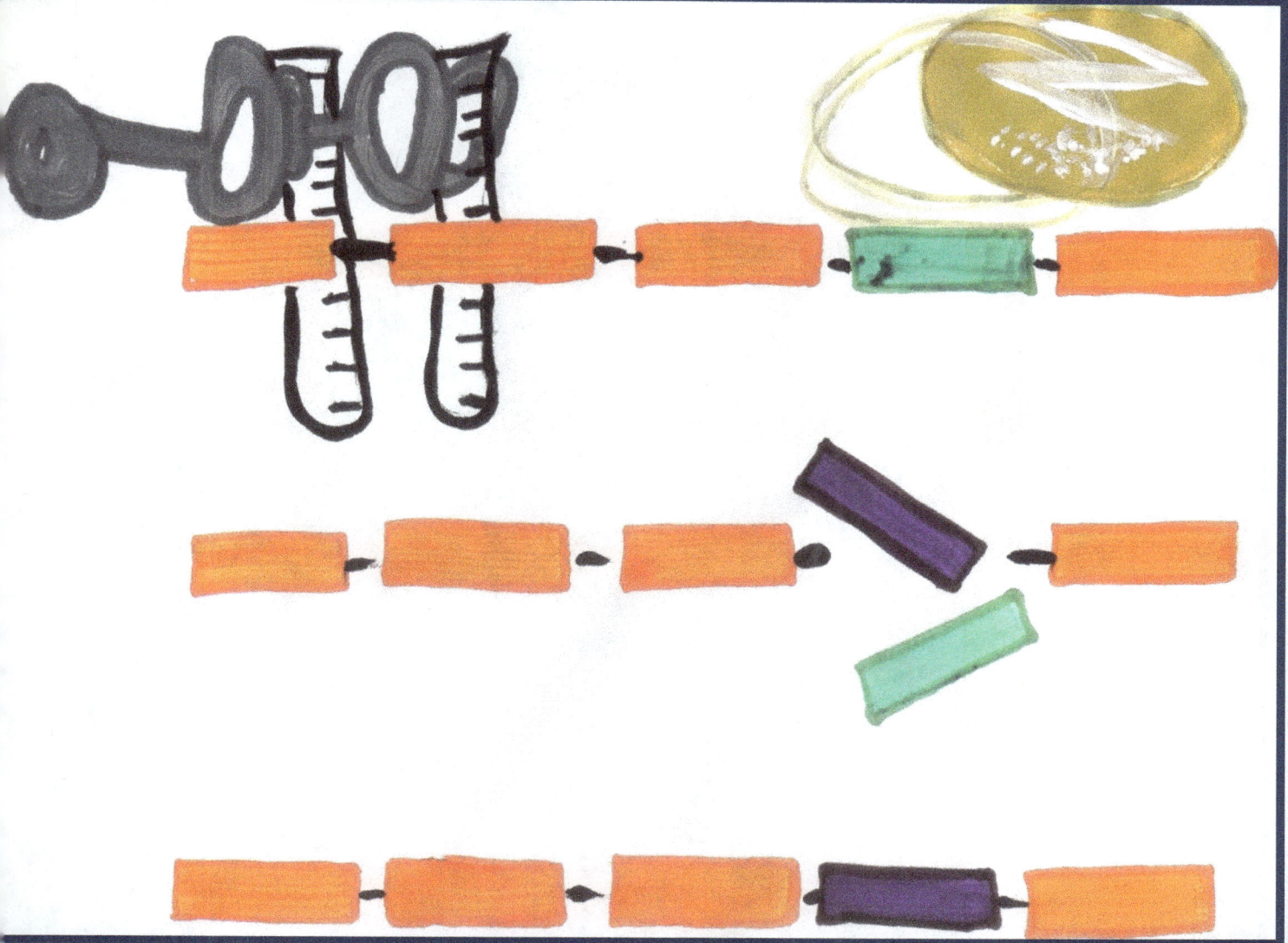

There are doctors of science testing genes in research to replace my gene that does not quite work.

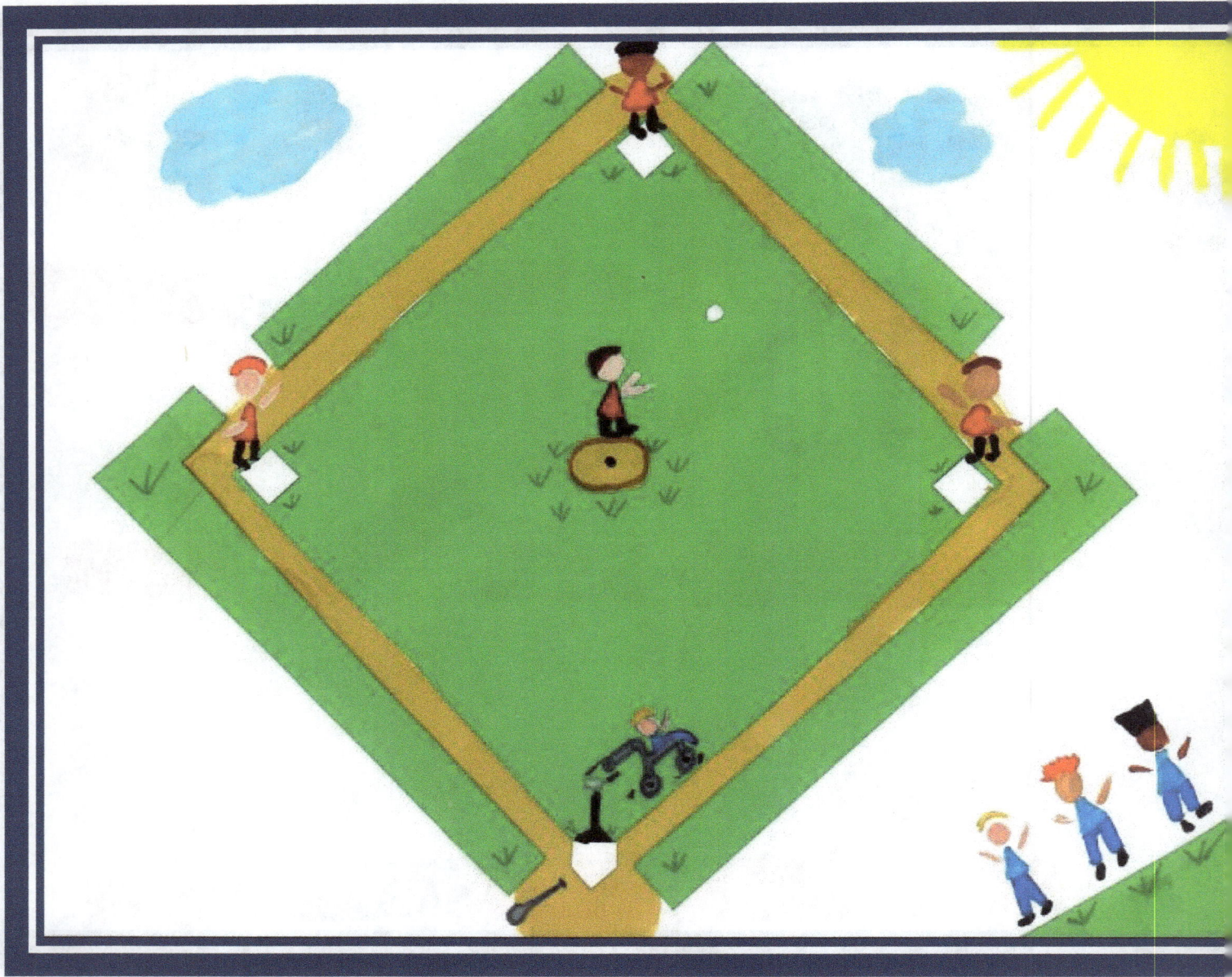

Do you know what truly makes my day?
It's when my friends find an imaginative way
to change or create a game so that I can play!

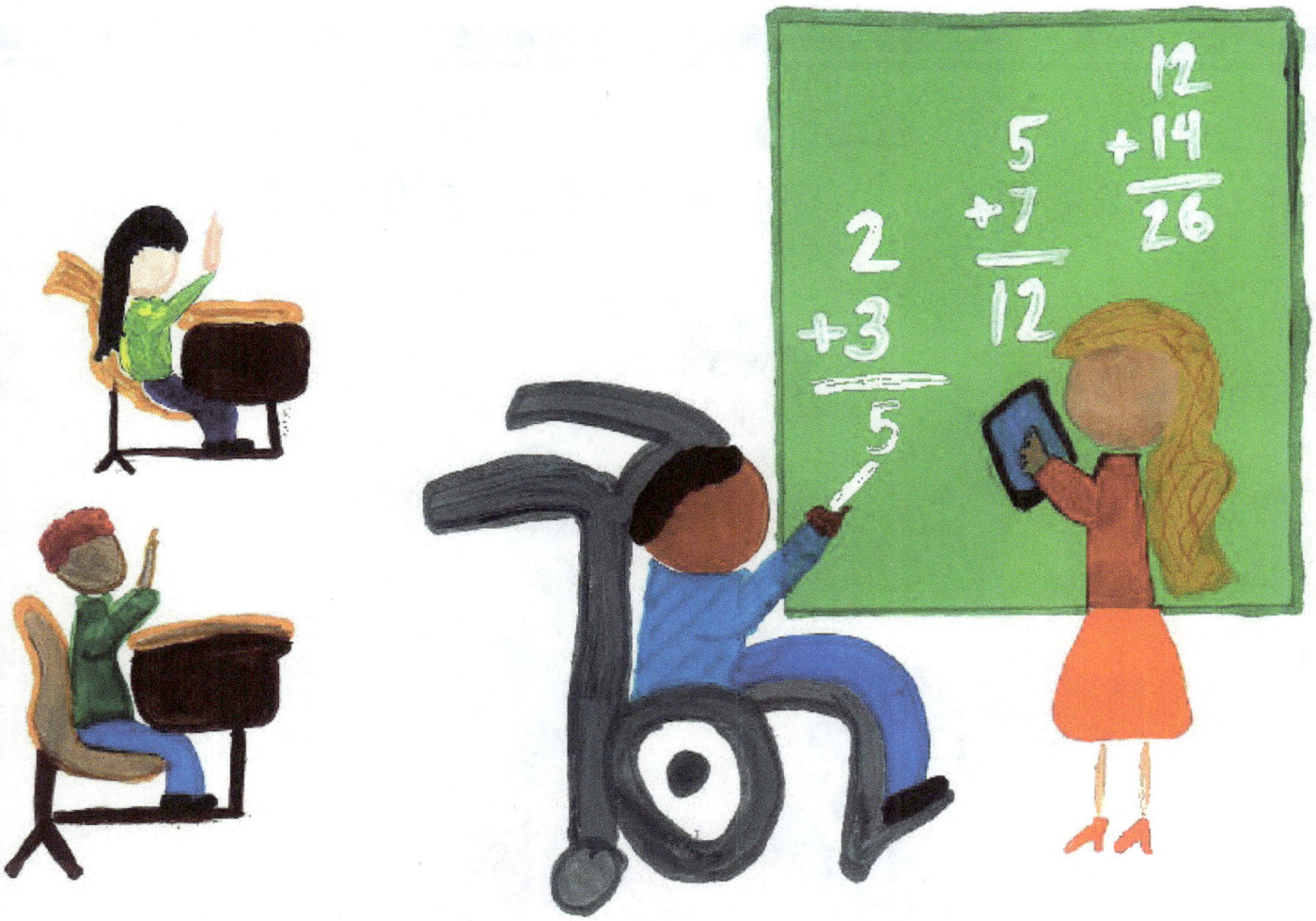

Another thing I think is cool
is when a teacher uses an innovative tool
to enhance my learning at school!

My parents join support groups to help us to cope.
Knowing other kids just like me gives me hope.

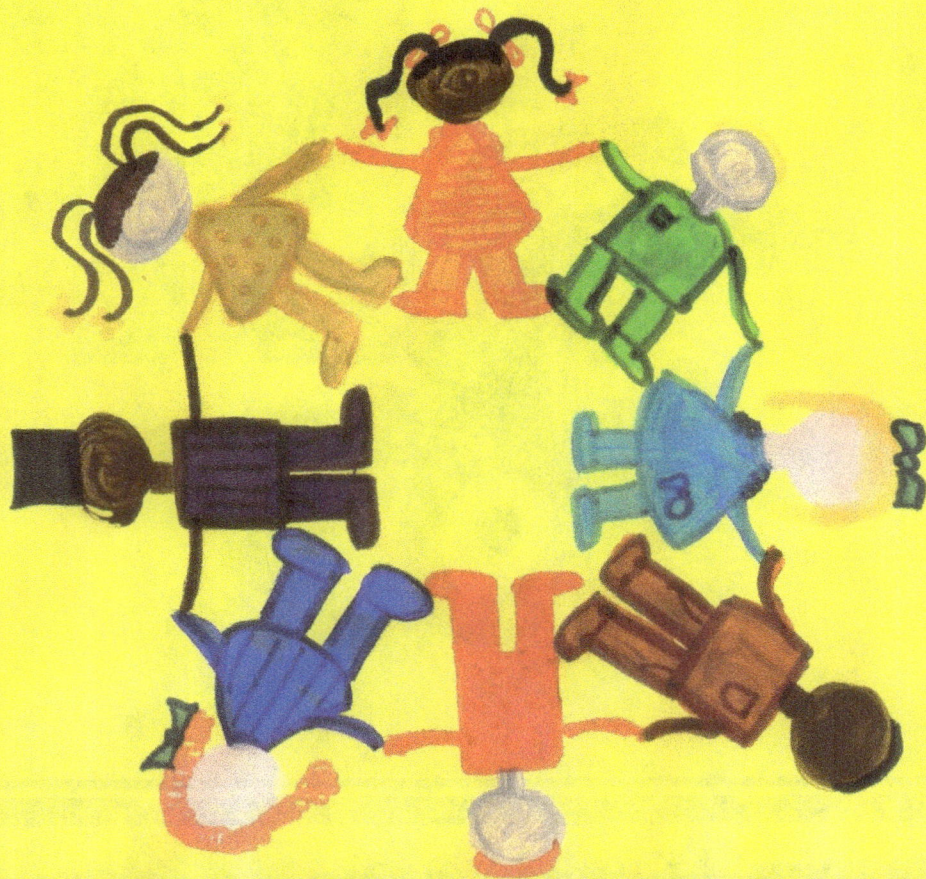

One day I believe I'll walk careless and free,
but until that day comes look beyond this and see
what a great child I am and just love me for me.

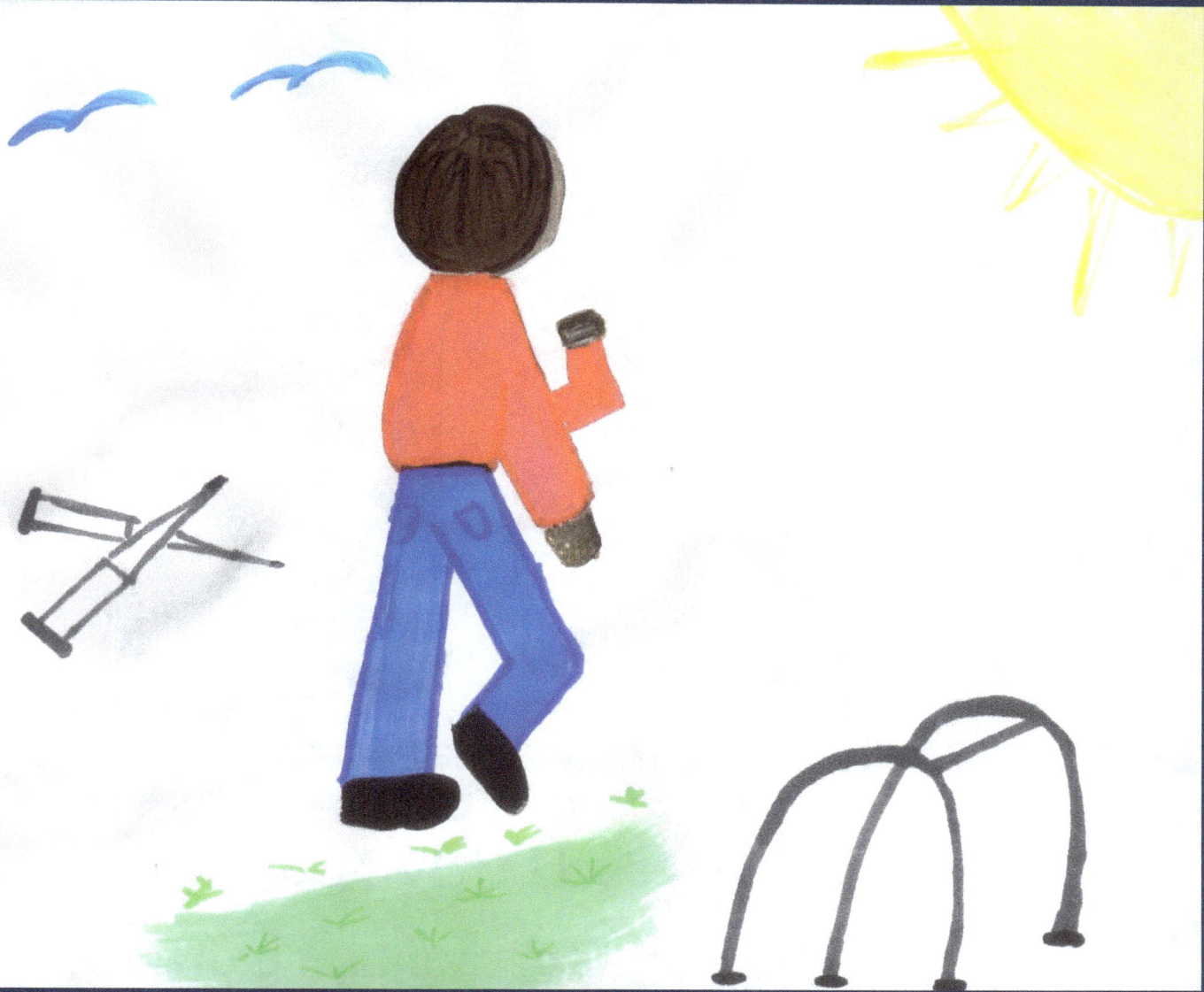

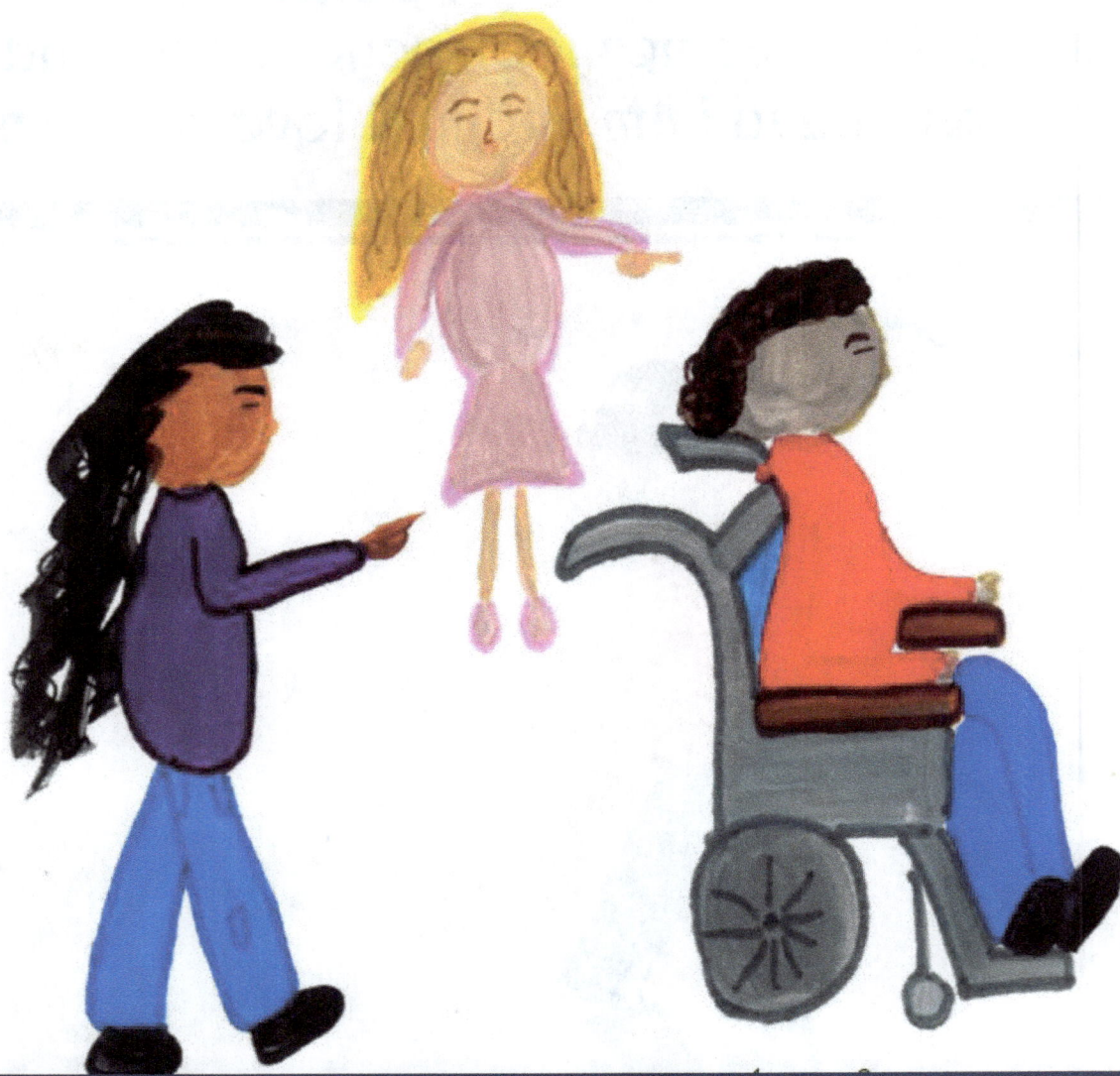

So if you see me in passing, don't point and stare, please! I HAVE Spinal Muscular Atrophy, but I am a person not a disease!

About Spinal Muscular Atrophy

▶ Spinal Muscular Atrophy (SMA) is a neuromuscular condition with an incidence in the United States of 1 in 6,000 to 10,000 children. There are nerves in the spinal cord and brainstem that do not work due to a gene defect. If these nerves do not work or progressively the nerve cells die, they are unable to send signals telling the muscles to contract. Therefore, the muscles become weak. Children with this condition generally have trouble sitting up, crawling and walking, and in some instances, even the muscles of respiration are affected, and patients may have difficulty breathing. Additionally, there may be problems with eating, swallowing, and digestion. There are 5 main types (SMA 0, I, II, III, & IV). They are due to a defect in the *SMN1* gene. However, there are several other less common forms of SMA that are caused by other genes. Children with SMA have a normal range of intelligence. It is important that educators find creative solutions to helping them learn in a supportive environment. 1 in 50 people in the population are considered carriers. This means that they have a mutated gene. If one person who is a carrier has a child with another person who is a carrier, that couple may have a child with SMA. All races may be affected, but Caucasians have a greater incidence.

▶ SMA does not have a cure, but many things are being done to treat the symptoms. Research is currently underway to replace the defective gene or faulty protein. These studies provide hope of cure in the near future.

References:

▶ Prior, T.W.; Russman, B.S., "Spinal Muscular Atrophy" GeneReviews ®. February 24, 2000. http://www.ncbi.nlm.nih.gov/books/NBK1352/ (accessed December 21, 2015).

▶ http://www.genome.gov/20519681 (accessed December 21, 2015).

For more information and support, visit:

▶ www.facebook.com/KureforKalen

▶ www.CureSMA.org

▶ www.renwillwalk.org

▶ http://ghr.nlm.nih.gov/condition/spinal-muscular-atrophy Genetics Home Reference, a service of the U.S. National Library of Medicine

▶ Medline Plus Spinal Muscular Atrophy

▶ National Library of Medicine Genetics Home Reference Spinal muscular atrophy

▶ National Organization for Rare Disorders (NORD) Email: RN@rarediseases.org; genetic_counselor@rarediseases.org; orphan@rarediseases.org Spinal Muscular Atrophy

- ▶ NCBI Genes and Disease Spinal muscular atrophy
- ▶ Claire Altman Heine Foundation, Inc. www.clairealtmanheinefoundation.org
- ▶ Muscular Dystrophy Association – USA (MDA) www.mda.org
- ▶ International SMA Patient Registry smaregistry.iu.edu

About the Author and
Inspiration for This Text

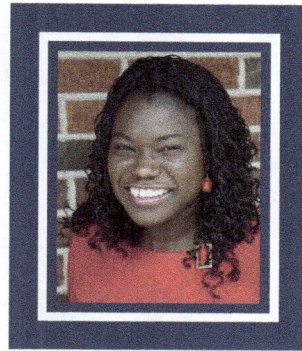

▶ **Christy L. Ott, MD** is a board-certified pediatrician currently practicing medicine at Family Health Services: Pediatric Healthcare Associates in the city of Chattanooga, TN. Inspired by the stories of Kyan and Kalen Kulas, two brothers who both were diagnosed with Spinal Muscular Atrophy Type 2 in early childhood, *One in Ten Thousand* is a story of courageous children who experience the challenges of SMA every day.

▶ *One in Ten Thousand* attempts to capture the emotions, questions, fears and hopes of children and families affected by SMA in a child-friendly format.

▶ With the incidence of SMA being 1/6,000- 1/10,000 children, the story is written with the intent to raise awareness, support and encourage families, and the profits will be shared with the Cure SMA foundation to promote research aims.

▶ Disclaimer from the author: Through humor this story alludes to God making a mistake or even God having SMA. It is not intended to suggest that God is fallible or that children with SMA are an accident, but rather to bring a smile as a child realizes that we have a God who understands our situation. Hebrews 4:15 says, "For we do not have a high priest who is unable to empathize with our weaknesses, but we have one who has been tempted in every way, just as we are—yet he did not sin." This verse suggests to me that God understands weakness, illness, and everything that makes us human. James 1:2 tells us to consider it a joy when we are given trials because it teaches us the character of patience. The children and families whom I have had the pleasure to encounter typically demonstrate joy and courage despite difficult life circumstances. I hope this story encourages kids not to give up and supports families in their quest for cures.

▶ Dr. Ott is also the author of a bedtime story entitled, *I Don't Like Night, Mommy!* To purchase her other works, visit www.christyott.com.

www.ingramcontent.com/pod-product-compliance
Lightning Source LLC
Chambersburg PA
CBHW081555220326
41598CB00036B/6682

* 9 780692 639283 *